MEN'S HEALTH BEST

WEIGHT-FREE WORKOUT

MEN'S HEALTH BEST

WEIGHT-FREE
WORKOUT

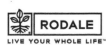
RODALE
LIVE YOUR WHOLE LIFE™

Every day our brands connect with and inspire millions of
people to live a life of the mind, body, spirit — a whole life.

Edited by Joe Kita, *Men's Health* Magazine

If you want to build muscle, improve your sex life, and do nearly everything better, visit our Web site at menshealth.com

© 2005 by Rodale Inc.

Cover photograph by Robert Wright

Interior photographs
Beth Bischoff p. 31, 32, 37, 38, 39, 42, 43, 48, 49, 50, 51, 64, 66, 67, 68, 69, 70, 71, 74, 76, 79, 84, 85, 86, 87, 88, 89, 90, 91, 92, 93, 94; Brand X Pictures p. 6, 33; Corbis p. 14, 21; Digital Vision p. 63; Todd France p. 34, 35, 40, 41; Svend Lindbaek p. 89; Michael Mazzeo p. 11, 22, 23, 24, 25, 26, 27, 28, 29, 30, 44, 45, 46, 47, 52, 53, 54, 55, 58, 59, 60, 61, 62, 65, 72, 73, 75, 77, 78, 80, 81, 82, 83; Photodisc p. 9, 16, 36.

Men's Health® is a registered trademark of Rodale Inc.

Printed in the United States of America.

Library of Congress Catalog-in-Publication data is on file with the publisher.
1–59486–259–1
Distributed to the book trade by Holtzbrinck Publishers
10 12 14 15 13 11 9 paperback

LIVE YOUR WHOLE LIFE™

We inspire and enable people to improve their lives and the world around them
For more of our products visit **rodalestore.com** or call 800-848-4735

CONTENTS

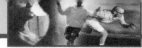

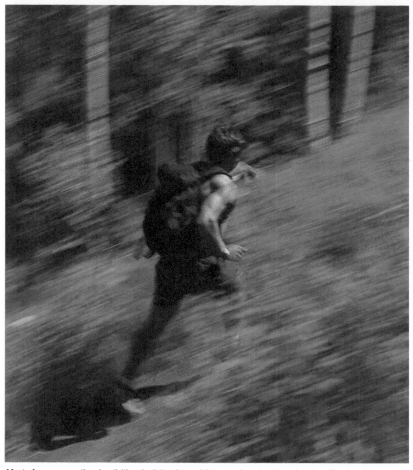

Most of your recreational activities don't involve weights—so knowing how to train without weights makes good sense.

INTRODUCTION

When we picture a modern-day workout we almost always picture a guy at the gym standing, sitting, or lying down at a machine stacked with weights. Although there's no arguing that weight training can be an important part of any man's fitness routine, there are many practical reasons why a weight-free workout can be just as effective, serve as an occasional alternative to weights, or actually be more beneficial for certain types of men, depending on their fitness goals.

First of all, a weight-free workout can be done almost anywhere. The classic excuse, "I don't have time to go to the gym," doesn't apply when you're working weight-free. Your gym can be your living room, your basement, or even your office. Research has shown that as little as 15 minutes a day in an effective, balanced workout can be immensely beneficial. So, who doesn't have 15 minutes each day to devote to working out weight-free wherever they might happen to be?

A weight-free workout can actually be necessary for some people who have suffered an injury. When your doctor has recommended a low-impact workout to limit stress on certain muscles or joints, or to help you recover from lower back pain, working out weight-free can be the right way to go because the resistance you use in a weight-free workout comes from your own muscles and body weight. You are not forcing yourself to deal with an unrealistic weight mass attached to a machine, dumbbell, or barbell.

A less obvious but increasingly understood element of working without weights has to do with the body's core and sense of balance. Research into the muscles of the lower back and abdomen, and studies of fast-twitch muscle fibers and such core muscles as the psoas have consistently found that weight-free activities such as Pilates, yoga, and plyometrics help to enhance people's ability to maintain proper balance, posture, and form, enabling them to move faster in quick bursts of energy when playing sports or working out. When you are standing, sitting, or lying at a weight machine, or trying to negotiate the weights attached to a dumbbell or barbell, you are working your muscles hard but not necessarily conditioning your lower back and abdominals to support your body most effectively.

The basic stretches and exercises that make up a weight-free workout will work every major muscle group in your body. We've supplied you with the definitive guide to some classic moves, such as the pushup, press, and crunch, as well as some you may not have heard of before

STAY HEALTHY

Researchers examined the absentee records of 79,000 workers at 250 sites and found that those who maintained a minimum of two 20-minute workouts a week had fewer sick days than those who didn't exercise at all.

(including such moves from the animal kingdom as Cat-Camel on page 38, Dirty Dog on page 92, and Donkey Kick on page 94). We've also researched the latest in diet and nutrition information to maximize your progress. Research increasingly reveals that food, the essential fuel that powers your workout (and the rest of your day), is a vital component in any fitness program. We'll give you the latest on carbohydrates (yes, there are good carbs), protein (perhaps the single most important solid food component for men working out and trying to lose weight), and how to satisfy your hunger while you're trimming fat and building muscle mass. You'll also get a rundown of the major muscles and how they relate to one another, because we believe that if you're going to make a disciplined weight-free workout routine a regular part of your life, you should understand exactly what parts of your body are being worked, why, and how you can prevent injuring yourself in the process.

A suggestion on how to read this book: We're not suggesting you don't know how to read, but we thought we'd point out that if you're a few weeks away from hitting the beach for the first time this year, or if you're training for a marathon and are dying to know how a weight-free workout can strengthen your legs, don't feel compelled to take in the entire book at once. Flip around (for instance, to "Lower-Body Beach Blast," page 48, or "Sculpt Olympian Legs," page 44) and find what interests you most.

Most of all, have fun. We've had a blast putting these workouts and information together for you, and we hope you'll enjoy yourself even more as you get to work on that new body of yours.

MEASURE UP

You're embarking on a new fitness program; this book is your road map. But to use a map properly you've got to know where you are and where you want to go. The solution: Measure everything. Your neck, chest, waist, arms, thighs, and calves. Write it all down and put it someplace where you'll have to look at it every day. Record your weight, too, although that's less important. Your goal: Maintain or reduce the size of your waist while increasing the size of everything else. Repeat your measurements every four weeks.

PART I:
The Weight-Free Way

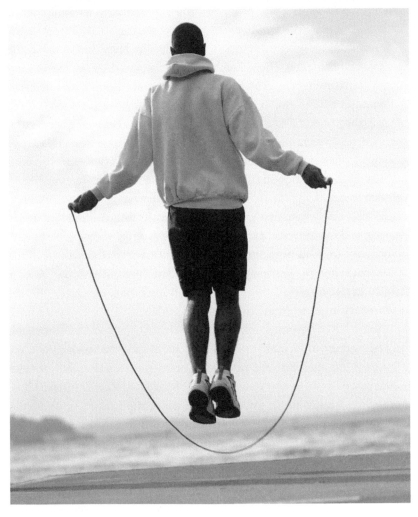

Weight-Free Workout Basics

The history of weight-free workouts would probably begin many millennia ago when our forebears discovered the value of putting their muscles through their paces. Back then, such workouts were more commonly known as "running for your life" or "defending your cave." Any way you look at it, weight-free has been around a lot longer than dumbbells, barbells, or any of the other finely calibrated machines in the modern-day gym. Today, weight-free means working your muscles by using your body weight, the force of gravity, and resistance created by props such as balls, blocks, and towels.

A weight-free workout might be done by a professional athlete between games in a hotel room, a business executive marooned at a conference center, or anyone who prefers to work out in the privacy of his home, office, or anywhere he can grab 10 minutes of time for himself.

A good mechanic understands every inch of a car's engine before he starts tinkering with it. Before you start overhauling your physique, you should have a working knowledge of the major muscle groups that power your body. Each one of the muscle groups described below (and indicated on the model at right) is addressed by one or more of the workouts that begin on page 33. The majority of the exercises referred to on the following pages can be found in Part III, beginning on page 63.

1. *Pectoralis major.* This large muscle, shaped like a fan, covers the front of the upper chest. A wide variety of pushups and the towel chest fly work the "pecs."

2. **Rhomboids.** Located in the middle of the upper back between the shoulder blades, the rhomboids are worked in exercises like pushups, the shoulder bridge, and the side straddle hop.

3. **Trapezius.** The "trap" is the upper part of the back, running from the back of the neck to the shoulders and is typically worked with pushups.

4. *Latissimus dorsi.* The much-sought-after "V" shape in the

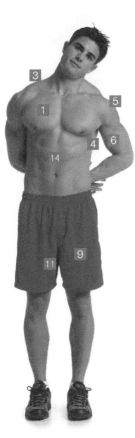

back comes from strong "lats." Pullups and chin-ups are great for working this group.

5. **Deltoids.** These muscles include the anterior deltoid, medial deltoid, and posterior deltoid and are located at the top of the shoulders. Pushups and the side straddle hop work the "delts."

6. **Biceps.** The front of the upper arms, the biceps group is the target of much weight training, much of it superfluous. Any

good exercise that involves the arms will work, but not overwork, the biceps.

7. **Triceps.** The back of the upper arm gets a good workout from a variety of pushups.

8. **Gluteals.** The "glutes" include the gluteus maximus, the muscle that covers your rear end. Lunges, squats, jumps, skips, stepups, and the shuttle run work the glutes.

9. **Quadriceps.** The "quads," a large muscle group, make up the front

FOLLOW THESE TWO SIMPLE EATING RULES

Finding time to exercise can be tough, especially when you have to adjust your workout to your eating schedule. Here's an easy to remember guide to pre- and postexercise nutrition (for a detailed look at diet and nutrition, see page 16):

1. Don't eat a big meal less than an hour before you work out, but do try to get something down before you exercise. Grab a carb-protein shake 5 minutes before your workout and sip on it throughout the session.

2. Eat carbohydrates and protein as soon as you can after your workout. The carbs help replace energy stores needed for your next workout; the protein repairs your muscles.

of the thigh. You'll work the quadriceps with lunges, squats, jumps, skips, and stepups.

10. **Hamstrings.** These large muscles run up the back of the thigh and need to be loose for almost any athletic activity. (You'll spend a good amount of time stretching your hamstrings before any workout.) Squats, jumps, skips, stepups, and the Shuttle Run especially target the hamstrings.

11. **Hip abductors and adductors.** These are the muscles of the inner and outer thigh. The abductors are located on the outside of your leg and move the leg away from the body. The adductors, located on the inside, pull the leg across the body. Exercises that work the hips include the Dirty Dog, Hip Adduction, and Donkey Kick.

12. **Calf.** Located on the back of the lower leg, the calf muscles include the *gastrocnemius* and the *soleus*. The *gastrocnemius* supplies the calf with its rounded shape. The *soleus* runs under the *gastrocnemius*. As with the hamstrings, you should devote some time to stretching the calf muscles, which are especially targeted by jumps, squats, skips, stepups, and the Shuttle Run.

13. **Lower back.** The *erector spinae* muscles support the back and are responsible for good posture (remember to work them next time someone tells you to stand up straight). Squats and floor exercises work the lower back.

14. Abdominals. The "abs" are made up of the *rectus abdominis*, which runs the length of the abdomen, and the external obliques, which are located on the sides and front of the abdomen. Crunches hit the *rectus abdominis*, and variations on the crunch such as twists work the external obliques. Boxing exercises such as the Horse-Stance Twist and "slip a punch," and floor exercises like the Curlup also work the abs.

Workout Basics

It seems that anything worth doing is worth making incredibly complicated, especially workouts. We start adding exercises to hit every muscle from every angle; we run forward, then backward, and sideways; we crunch, reverse crunch, side crunch, and numbers crunch. Then we're so confused we forget why we were working out in the first place. Drop the slide rule. It's time to make exercise simple again. Cut time, aggravation, and wasted effort without sacrificing results. You'll enjoy your weight-free routine more and profit more from it—which is why you work out in the first place, right?

Time of Day. Research has consistently shown that exercising at the same time each workout day increases your chances of sticking with it. Pick the time you like. You may have heard that morning workouts are better, since testosterone levels are higher. Now forget you heard that. Hormonal fluctuations are important, but they may not correlate to performance gains. The optimal time to work out is any time you can fit it into your schedule.

STRETCH

Nobody wants to be called a stiff. "Inflexible" and "rigid" are just as undesirable. A stiff body is like a trial separation from your well-being. Tight hamstrings can lead to runner's knee. Tight pectorals limit your strength and put your shoulders at risk of injury. We've included a number of vital stretches as part of the weight-free workout. Spend twice as much time stretching your tight muscles as your flexible muscles. You should focus on problem areas instead of muscles that are already flexible. If you're under 40, hold your stretches for 30 seconds. If you're over 40, hold them for 60 seconds. As you reach your 40s, your muscles become less pliable, so they need to be stretched longer.

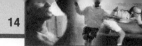

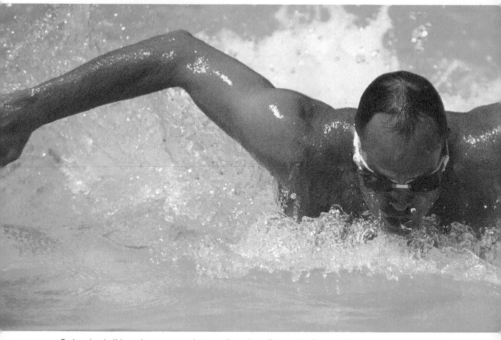

Swimming builds endurance, muscle strength, and cardiovascular fitness without stressing your body.

Keep a Calendar. Do the workout, and then cross it off. Mark an "X" on your calendar on the days you exercise. A recent study found that exercisers who used this simple system of tracking workouts made more progress than those who didn't.

Stick With It. Stay with an exercise program until it stops working for you. Switching too often from one program to the next can get in the way of your goals. You'll make your workouts simpler (and see better results) if you stick to one program for six to 12 weeks, or until it quits working. Is it working? Two

benchmarks: Your waist tightens while your strength improves.

One at a Time. Do one exercise for each muscle group. Unless you're a bodybuilder, there's no need to hit a muscle from every conceivable angle each time you train it. Work hard on one or two exercises per muscle group.

Set a Time Limit. Forget the hours of working out you imagine other guys are doing. Aim for one hour. The dropout rate for routines that last more than 60 minutes is high. At one hour, your body slows down its production of muscle-

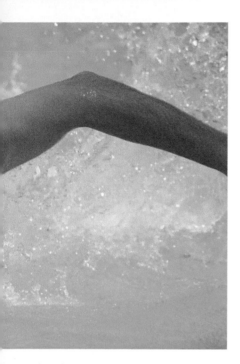

Reach Your Goals. Set your goals in reverse. That is, pick a date of completion and work backward, writing down short-term goals as you go. The goals then seem more like deadlines.

Stay Hydrated. Start the day with a liter bottle of water. Finish it off by the end of the day. Along with other beverages like milk and juice, that should keep you hydrated. Alcohol doesn't count—it not only makes you sprint to the urinal, it takes some of your body's own water out, too.

Drinking too much alcohol can lower your testosterone levels and decrease overall muscle mass. However, drinking moderately (two drinks or less per day) won't harm testosterone levels and can actually improve your cardiovascular health.

Sleep. Depriving yourself of sleep not only limits your ability to grow muscle—your body releases most of its growth hormone while you sleep—but also severely impairs your coordination and mental focus. This translates to less strength and a greater chance of injuring yourself. If you work out, you should sleep for the optimum amount of time each night—at least seven or eight hours a night for most guys. If you have to go a few nights with limited sleep, don't count on your best performance.

building hormones and cranks up the stress hormone cortisol, which can have a testosterone-blocking, muscle-wasting effect.

Recover Faster. A lot of people adopt a weight-free workout because they've sustained an injury that requires a low-impact fitness routine. If you're recovering from a muscle injury, begin exercising again as soon as you can. Try a few minutes at low intensity to test yourself. Go slowly— no explosive movements. If you experience pain, stop immediately. Afterward, ice the area for 20 minutes and exercise again the next day. You should be able to go a little harder and longer each workout.

Diet and Nutrition

You're going to get hungry every two to three hours, guaranteed. Whatever your fitness goals, whatever the frequency and intensity of your workouts, the key to diet and nutrition is: Be prepared. If you know you're going to be away from decent food, take some healthy snacks with you. Nuts and dried fruit are easy and compact, and require no special preparation or refrigeration. If you need to pack something more meal-like, try a peanut butter and jelly sandwich on whole-grain bread. Keep apples nearby everywhere you go; if you make it through one apple a day, the pectin will keep you too full to crave anything really awful.

Protein

A recent study compared high carbohydrate with high protein diets for weight loss in extremely overweight men. Even though the calories were the same, the high protein group lost 28 percent more weight in the four week study. More importantly, the metabolic rates of the men in the high protein group were 14 percent higher than the others. Try eating around one gram of protein per pound of body weight. Any excess will be stored as fat.

Unfortunately, shopping for, preparing, and eating that much protein

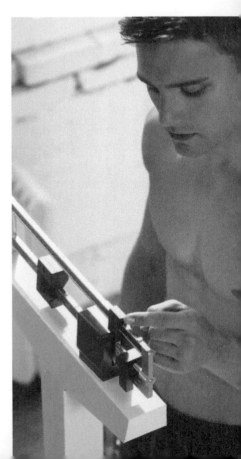

Add the right exercises to your weight-loss plan to ensure you don't diet away all that hard-earned muscle.

could turn into a part-time job, which explains the popularity of protein-based meal replacement supplements. A single serving of a typical supplement contains between 18 and 40 grams of protein. All are sweetened with a sugar called maltodextrin, so you don't have to add anything but water and then mix them up in a shaker or blender. Two servings can supply your daily protein allowance.

Protein bars are another alternative, with one minor drawback. Many are often made with chemicals called sugar alcohols, and too much of these in your system can lead to serious flatulence. You shouldn't experience this problem if you keep your intake to one bar a day—but consider yourself warned.

Carbohydrates

The best carbohydrates for your metabolism are those with a low glycemic index. The glycemic index measures how fast your body processes a food. Foods with a high index (such as white bread and highly processed breakfast cereals) make you hungrier faster.

Unfortunately, there's nothing intuitive about the glycemic index. Many people consider pasta to be a fast acting carbohydrate, but most pastas fall in the middle of the range. And a high fiber cereal like shredded wheat is near the top.

In other words, if you want to use the glycemic index, you have to spend time memorizing it, or use a cheat sheet. The box below shows how to replace five common high

GLYCEMIC SWAP LIST

Foods with a low glycemic index are slow burners, so they'll keep you full longer. A simple rule for slowing your body's response to food, no matter how high the glycemic index, is to add protein, fat, and/or fiber to any meal. The glycemic index numbers following the foods in this chart are based on a scale on which pure glucose has a score of 100. The higher the number, the faster the food burns.

Instead of...	Try...
White bread (70)	Mixed-grain bread (48)
Corn flakes (83)	Bran cereal (58)
Baked potato (85)	Protein-enriched spaghetti (27)
Watermelon (72)	Pear (37)
Chocolate-caramel bar (64)	Peanut-based candy (32)

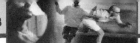

SOURCES OF PROTEIN

Food	Protein (grams)
6-oz chicken breast, cooked weight	52
2 slices (6-oz) lean roast beef, cooked weight	49
6-oz can of tuna	41
roast beef sandwich	22
6 egg whites	21
turkey sandwich on wheat bread	18
2 whole eggs	13
1 cup baked beans	12
8-oz container of low fat yogurt	11
1/2 cup cashews, or about 40 to 50 nuts	11
1 cup spaghetti, cooked	7
1 cup oatmeal	5
1 cup fat-free milk	1

glycemic foods with others that are lower on the list.

Perfect Meal Timing

If you want to understand energy balance in an instant, think of your body as a car that operates 24 hours a day. You would never expect your car to get you from one place to the next without systematic refueling, just as you know there's no point in putting more gas in the tank than it's designed to hold, but that's how many of us operate our bodies. We try to run on empty for hours, then dump in more fuel than we can handle. This strategy is self-destructive.

Let's say you really want to lose fat, and decide to jog first thing in the morning on an empty stomach. The easiest way to get energy is to break down muscle mass. Your body can convert specific amino acids— the building blocks of muscle—to glucose, the sugar that powers human activity. Someone running before eating may actually be breaking down the very tissue he's trying to improve. This is counterproductive—a "muscle-loss" diet.

The "fat-gain" diet is probably more typical of most of us. With this one, you wait a long time between meals, and then, when you're ravenously hungry, you wipe out an entire buffet line. This guarantees that you'll get a larger surge of the hormone insulin than you ordinarily would and that means more fat storage.

You can probably combine the "muscle-loss" and "fat-gain" strategies mentioned about to turn your body into a perfect muscle-burning, fat-storing machine. Hard exercise slows down appetite in the short term, but as you get used to it, your appetite matches your exertion level. So you go out and run 10 miles on an empty stomach, then eat enough to fuel a 15-mile run, the net effect is that you've lost muscle on the run and gained fat from the postrun meal. Energy balance is the answer:

- Eat as soon as you wake up.

- Make sure you eat a small meal before you exercise, no matter what time of day it is. Not only does the food prevent your muscle tissue from becoming cardio chow, it also increases the number of calories you burn during and after exercise. Studies show that exercise following a meal enhances metabolism.

- Eat immediately after exercising, when your body has depleted its energy reserves. Act fast, or you'll start burning muscle for energy.

- Eat a total of five to six small meals each day. Studies have shown that athletes who added three daily snacks to their three square meals lost fat and gained muscle, besides improving in all the other things that are important to athletes, such as

SHAKE YOUR MUSCLES

Eat immediately after your workout. A recent Danish study (the country, not the pastry) found that older men who drank a shake with 10 grams of protein, 7 grams of carbohydrate, and 3 grams of fat (about the same as in a cup of milk) within five minutes after their weight workout gained muscle, but men who consumed the drink two hours later did not. For a serious postworkout muscle-building shake, try this formula:

Blend a half-cup of fat-free frozen chocolate yogurt, a quarter-cup of egg substitute, a cup of fat-free milk, a large banana, and a tablespoon of unsweetened cocoa powder, and drink. You'll down 23 grams of protein, 52 grams of carbs, and only four grams of fat.

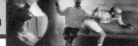
WORKOUT MEAL PLAN

Use this great meal-planning system when your exercise affects what you should eat, and when you should eat it.

IF YOU WORK OUT IN THE MORNING

Meal 1: PREWORKOUT SNACK

- 1/2 whey protein shake (or)
- banana and hard-boiled egg (or)
- cereal with fat-free milk

Meal 2: BREAKFAST

(Immediately following workout)

- egg-white omelette with vegetables, and oatmeal
- orange juice

Meal 3: MIDMORNING SNACK

- yogurt and fruit (or)
- whey protein shake and fruit

Meal 4: LUNCH

- salad with grilled chicken and olive oil dressing (or) tuna or lunchmeat sandwich on whole-grain bread

Meal 5: MIDAFTERNOON SNACK

- peanut butter or cashews and an apple (or)
- meal-replacement bar (or)
- jerky

Meal 6: DINNER

- grilled salmon, chicken breast, or sirloin steak
- green salad with olive oil dressing

IF YOU WORK OUT AT LUNCH

Meal 1: BREAKFAST

- scrambled eggs with whole-grain toast (or)
- oatmeal with crushed flaxseeds and yogurt

Meal 2: MIDMORNING/PREWORKOUT SNACK

(No more than one hour before workout)

- whey protein shake with fruit

Meal 3: LUNCH

(Immediately following workout)

- chicken breast sandwich on kaiser roll
- fruit

Meal 4: MIDAFTERNOON SNACK

- peanut butter or cashews and an apple (or)
- meal-replacement bar (or)
- jerky

Meal 5: DINNER

- Hamburger made with ground sirloin (90% lean) or turkey on whole-grain bun
- cucumber-tomato salad drizzled with olive oil

IF YOU WORK OUT RIGHT AFTER WORK

Meal 1: BREAKFAST
- scrambled eggs with whole-grain toast (or)
- whole-grain cereal with blueberries and skim milk

Meal 2: MIDMORNING SNACK
- whey protein shake with peanut butter (or)
- yogurt and cashews

Meal 3: LUNCH
- chicken breast
- steamed vegetables
- roll

Meal 4: MIDAFTERNOON SNACK
- peanut butter or cashews and an apple (or)
- meal-replacement bar (or)
- jerky

Meal 5: PREWORKOUT SNACK
- 1/2 whey protein shake

Meal 6: DINNER
- grilled salmon, chicken breast, or sirloin steak
- green salad with olive oil dressing
- wild rice

power and endurance. Of course, you can't simply add a few hundred calories to your diet and lose weight, but you can redistribute your daily calories so you're eating more often but consuming less at individual meals.

- Eat before bed. If you're trying to build muscle and lose fat, you may need to eat right before bed to keep your body from breaking down muscle tissue as you sleep. Planning this snack will help you resist the temptation to inhale an entire chocolate cake at midnight.

However you do it, it's clear that the worst dieting strategy is cutting out tons of calories indiscriminately in hopes of sudden dramatic weight loss. If you're more patient and try to lose a pound a week every week or two, you'll be more likely to reach your goals and less likely to regain those unwanted pounds.

The Benefits of Stretching

Some men are so crunched for time that they just want to get their workout over with as quickly as possible. They just want to get right into it without warming up or stretching before they begin. But just a few minutes of stretching can be enormously beneficial to your workout. Just five to seven minutes of stretching before and after exercise will increase flexibility. Stretching prevents injury and soreness, helps free your body of muscular tension, improves circulation, and enhances muscle tone—giving your muscles a more defined look.

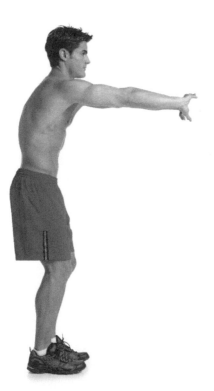

UPPER-BACK STRETCH

Hold your arms straight out in front of your chest and clasp your hands together. Push your arms forward, rounding your shoulders and upper back. Hold for 10 seconds.

CHEST STRETCH

Clasp your hands together, palms up, behind your lower back. Pull your arms up toward your head. Hold 10 seconds. Feel the stretch in the front of your chest and shoulders.

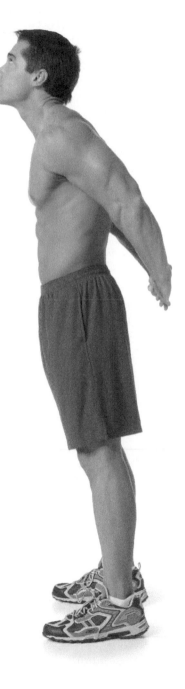

SHOULDER AND NECK STRETCH

Place both arms behind your back and grab your right wrist with your left hand. Tilt your head to the left and pull your right arm to the left. Hold for 10 seconds, then repeat on the other side.

HOW OFTEN SHOULD I STRETCH?

If you're stuck behind a desk all day, stretch every few hours to avoid back and shoulder tightness that comes from hunching over a keyboard. Do the Chest Stretch on page 23 to open your chest and relax your shoulders and back. To stretch your glued-to-the-chair glutes, cross your left leg over your right, resting your left ankle on your right knee. Bend forward at the waist and hold the stretch for 10 seconds. Then switch legs and repeat.

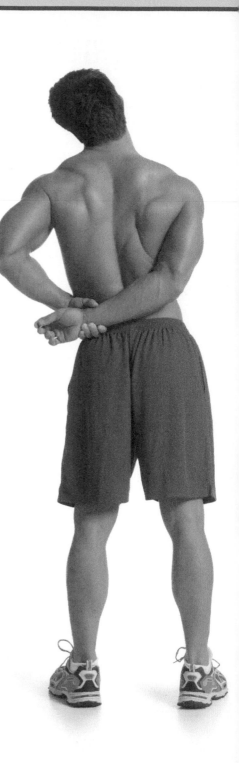

POSTERIOR SHOULDER STRETCH

Grab the back of your left upper arm with your right hand and pull it across your chest gently. Hold for 10 seconds, then repeat on the other side.

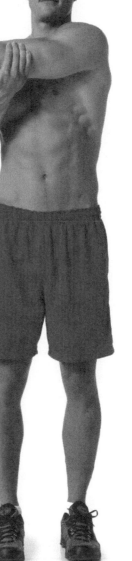

Towel Stretch Circuit

Your muscles, like a good after-dinner glass of brandy, work best when warm. That's why you can do more challenging stretches at the end of a workout without much risk of injury.

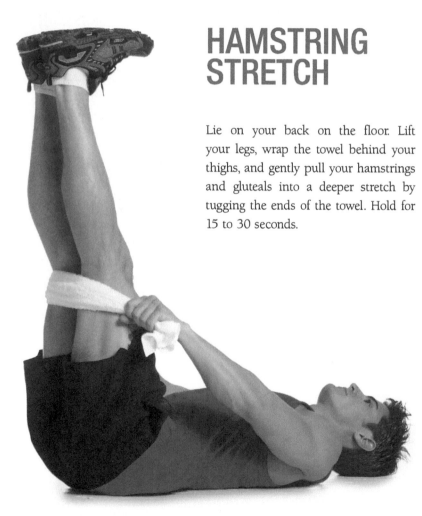

HAMSTRING STRETCH

Lie on your back on the floor. Lift your legs, wrap the towel behind your thighs, and gently pull your hamstrings and gluteals into a deeper stretch by tugging the ends of the towel. Hold for 15 to 30 seconds.

CHEST AND SHOULDER STRETCH

Now stand up, with the towel in your hands behind you. Bend forward as you reach back with your arms, slowly stretching out your chest and shoulders. Hold this position for 15 to 30 seconds.

WARM MUSCLES WORK BETTER

When muscles are cold, they're stiffer. Light exercise before stretching warms them and makes them more pliable, improving the stretch and reducing the risk of muscle strain. Keep it simple—walk or slowly jog for 10 minutes to prepare your muscles for the exercises ahead.

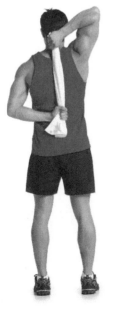

TRICEPS STRETCH

Finally, hold one end of the towel in your right hand and lift your right arm over your right shoulder, so the towel hangs down your back. Reach up behind you with your left hand and grab the other end of the towel. Gently pull your triceps and lats into a deeper stretch. Hold for 15 to 30 seconds, then repeat on the other side.

LYING ILIOTIBIAL BAND STRETCH

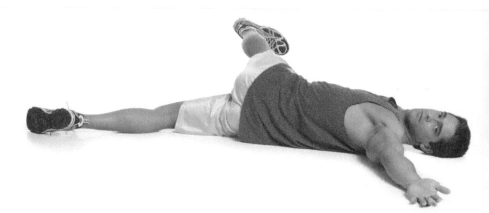

Lie on your back. Keep your left leg straight and lift it across your body.
Hold for 10 seconds. Repeat with the other leg.

BE FLEXIBLE

Flexibility is the easiest fitness element to develop. As with other types of training, improve-
ment in flexibility depends on subjecting muscles to more than they're accustomed to by
working them through a range of motion in a controlled and systematic way. You merely
need to add 10 extra minutes or so to what you already do.

MODIFIED HURDLER STRETCH

Sit on the floor with your left leg straight out in front of you. Place your right foot flat against your left thigh. Bend forward toward your left knee and hold for 10 seconds. Repeat with your right leg straight.

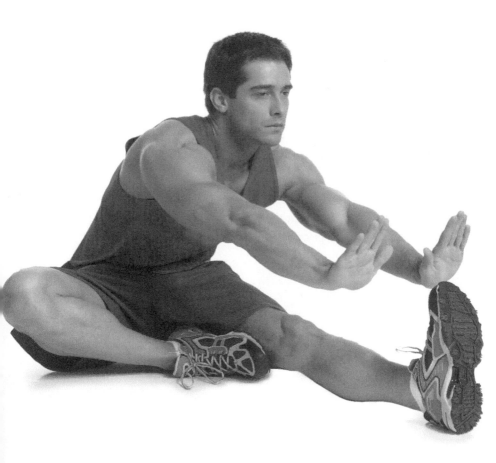

GROIN STRETCH

Sit on the floor and place the soles of your feet together. Grasp your ankles and gently push your knees down with your elbows. Hold for 10 seconds.

CALF STRETCH

From a standing position, step 2 feet forward with your left foot and bend your right knee. Bend at the waist, grab the front of your left foot, and pull it gently upward. (If necessary, place your free hand on a chair or wall for balance.) Hold for 10 seconds. Switch sides and repeat.

Full-Body Flexibility

Flexibility doesn't have to mean stretching and yoga and inner peace. It can mean sweat and grunts and a heart-pounding workout. These moves will stretch your muscles in ways that will help you with real-world activities, like starting a lawn mower. Perform these exercises as a circuit—one set of each stretch immediately after the other—as fast as possible. Do four or five circuits, 20 repetitions of each exercise. Two or three circuits is a good warmup for sports or weight lifting.

ROTATIONAL PRESS

Targets: Shoulders, Abdominals, Obliques, Gluteals, Calves, Ankles

Lift your right arm as high as you can above your shoulder and twist your body 90 degrees to the left, lifting your right heel as you turn. Then lower your right arm and raise your left arm as you twist to the right.

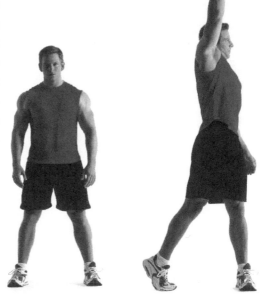

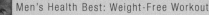

ALTERNATING UPRIGHT ROW

Targets: Lower Back, Chest, Obliques

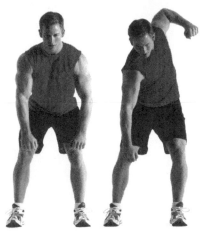

Bend over slightly at the hips until your upper body is at a 30-degree angle from vertical. Look at the floor and let your arms hang straight down from your shoulders. Then lift your left elbow as high as possible, as if starting a lawn mower. As you lower your left arm, repeat the movement with your right arm.

REACHING LATERAL LUNGE

Targets: Lower Back, Gluteals, Hamstrings

Step to the left with your left leg, keeping the toes of your left foot pointing forward. Bend your left knee about 20 degrees and bend over to touch the toes of your left foot with the fingertips of both hands. Push back to the starting position, then reach as high as you can with both hands. Repeat the movement to your right side. That's one repetition.

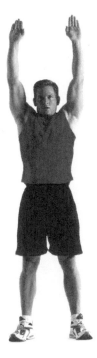

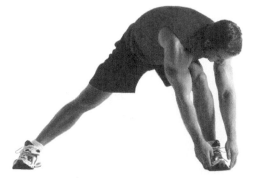

PART II:
Ultimate Workouts

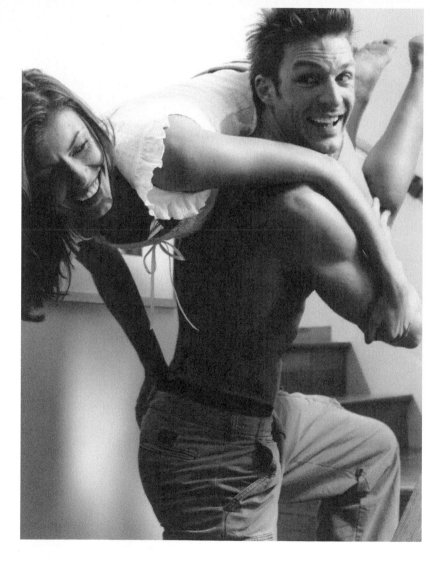

🕐 THE 15-MINUTE WORKOUT

Go to Extremes

The following three-step program might not be a 15-minute workout the first time you try it. It may take a few weeks to build up to that. Once you reach that point, you can add weight to make the moves even more difficult, try the exercises from different angles, or invent your own exercises using the techniques described here. Do this workout 3 days in a row, resting a day, doing it 2 more days, then resting 2 days. Repeat for the rest of your life, if you want.

EXTREME-RANGE ONE-LEG SQUAT

Targets: Quadriceps, Gluteus Maximus
Time: 5 Minutes

1. Stand with your back to a box, place your right foot on it, and squat down. Hold for 2 seconds then release.

2. Now, squat down farther and hold the position as long as you can bear the burn. Repeat until your leg can't take it anymore. Then repeat with your left foot on the box.

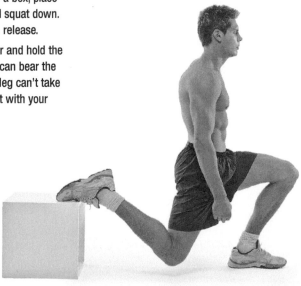

EXTREME-RANGE PULLUP

Targets: Biceps, Latissimus Dorsi, Trapezius
Time: 5 Minutes

1. Using an overhand grip with your arms just beyond shoulder width, hang from a pullup bar for 2 seconds. Drop from the bar and relax.

2. Now grab the bar again and hang as long as you can. Drop and rest a minute, then go up and hold again. Repeat until your back refuses to do any more.

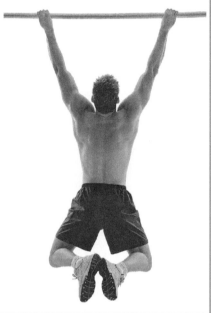

EXTREME-RANGE PUSHUP

Targets: Biceps, Latissimus Dorsi, Trapezius
Time: 5 Minutes

1. Set two sturdy boxes 30 to 36 inches apart. Drop into a pushup position and lower your chest between the boxes for 2 seconds.

2. Relax, then repeat, holding as long as you can. Rest a minute, then go down and hold again. Repeat until your upper body begs for mercy.

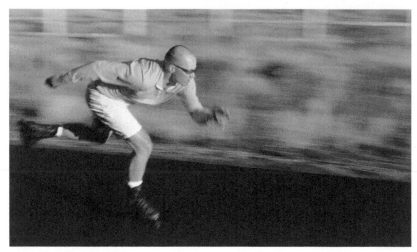

Strong lower-back muscles and powerful abdominals that stabilize your torso will help prevent lower-back strain when you rollerblade.

Save Your Back in 7 Minutes

Here is a back-saving program that not only relieves current back pain, but also reduces your chances of a future back attack. This quick and easy four-exercise circuit is designed to increase back strength and flexibility through endurance-building movements that will help stabilize your back muscles. The result: strong, supple back muscles that will support you during any activity—anytime, anywhere.

YOUR WORKOUT SCHEDULE

Do the workout once a day, every day. You don't need rest days between lower-back workouts, since the idea is to build endurance, rather than strength. Plus, by performing these exercises daily, you'll strengthen your spine-stabilizing muscles. Perform the exercises as a circuit, doing them consecutively without rest in between.

CURLUP

Targets: Entire Abdominal Region

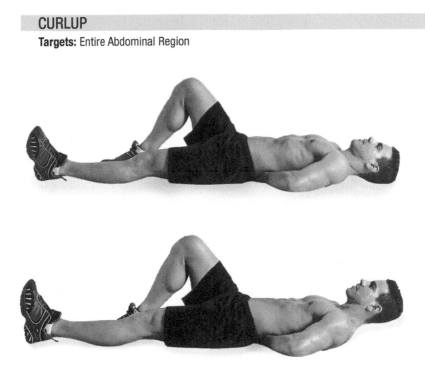

1. Lie faceup on the floor with your left leg straight and flat on the floor. Your right knee should be bent and your right foot flat. Place your hands palms down on the floor underneath the natural arch in your lower back (don't flatten your back).

2. Slowly raise your head and shoulders off the floor without bending your lower back or spine, and hold this position for 7 to 8 seconds, breathing deeply the entire time.

3. That's one repetition. Do four repetitions, then switch legs so that your right leg is straight and your left is bent.

TRAINER'S TIPS

- This exercise forces you to work all of your abdominal muscles while keeping your lower back in its naturally arched position. The move minimizes stress on your spine while increasing the endurance of the muscles.

- For a more challenging workout, try raising your elbows off the floor as you curl up, or begin the movement by contracting your abs, and then curl up against that force.

CAT-CAMEL

Targets: Trapezius, Pectorals, Spinal Erectors

1. Get down on your hands and knees with your hands shoulder-width apart. Slowly lower your head between your arms as you push up as high as you can with your back, rounding your spine.

2. When you reach the top of the movement, slowly lower your back as you lift your head up, extend your neck forward and up, and arch your lower back by moving your belly button toward the floor.

3. That's one repetition. Do five to eight repetitions.

POSTURE IS KEY

The most dangerous position for your spine is fully flexed, or bent forward like the letter C. Avoid that position by keeping your lower back in its naturally arched alignment in any exercise that requires you to bend over. Back injuries are common, but can be avoided through care and practice.

SIDE BRIDGE

Targets: Lateral Stabilizers

1 Lie on your left side with your knees straight and your upper body propped up on your left elbow and forearm. Place your right hand on your left shoulder and slowly raise your hips until your body forms a straight line from your shoulders to your knees.

2 Hold this position for 7 to 8 seconds, breathing deeply the entire time. Do four or five repetitions, then switch to your right side.

BIRD DOG

Targets: Lower- and Middle-Back Extensors

1 Get down on your hands and knees with your palms flat on the floor, shoulder-width apart. Slowly raise and straighten your right leg and left arm at the same time. Hold that position for 7 to 8 seconds, breathing deeply throughout the exercise.

2 Lower your arm and leg straight down, and then sweep them along the floor back into the starting position.

3 That's one repetition. Perform four repetitions, then switch sides.

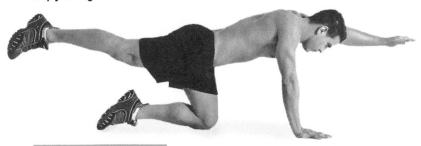

TRAINER'S TIP

This exercise works your lower- and middle-back extensors—the muscles that help you bend backward—while producing half the stress on your spine that conventional back-extension exercises create.

THE 15-MINUTE WORKOUT

Shadowbox For Ripped Abs

Boxers can tell you that great abs don't just look good: These muscles contract to protect your internal organs from body shots, and help you twist or lean to one side or the other to dodge fists or feet. That's why these modified boxing and martial-arts moves will help you build killer abs.

EXHALE AND CLENCH

Targets: Lateral Stabilizers
Time: 5 Minutes

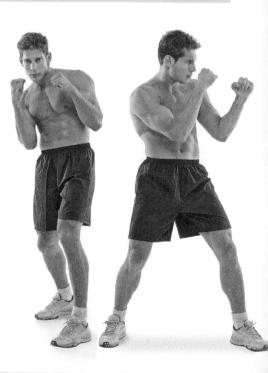

1. Stand in a boxing pose (one foo slightly in front of the other, han up) and imagine that you're absorbing a series of hits to the stomach.
2. Exhale and pull your belly in on each imagined strike.
3. Release your abdominal muscle and repeat.

TRAINER'S TIP

This exercise is great for your tran abdominis, the strip of muscle that ports your internal organs and flatt your waistline.

HORSE-STANCE TWIST

Targets: Obliques, Abdominals
Time: 5 Minutes

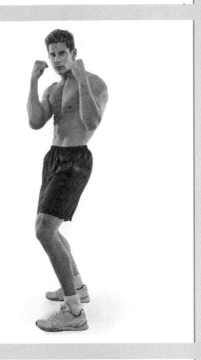

1. Stand with your feet just slightly beyond shoulder-width apart, toes pointed forward, knees bent at about a 60-degree angle, back straight, abs tight, hands up in a fighting posture.

2. Turn your torso to your left, pivoting on the balls of your feet if you need to (it's best to do this on an uncarpeted floor).

3. Feel the squeeze in the sides of your waist, then repeat to your right.

SLIP A PUNCH

Targets: Obliques, Abdominals
Time: 5 Minutes

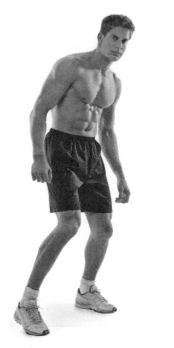

1. Start in the same position as the Horse-Stance Twist, only stand more upright, with your hands at your sides.

2. Imagine a punch is coming right at your nose (or get a trusted friend to actually throw one). Lean to the left just far enough to elude the punch. Don't move anything but your upper torso.

3. Feel that contraction on the left side of your waist? Now dodge a punch by leaning in the other direction.

Six-Pack Isolation

The exercises in this simple gut-busting workout are specifically designed to exhaust the oblique muscles first so your *rectus abdominis*—the six-pack—is isolated later. Perform this workout as a circuit, with no rest between exercises. Do three circuits, resting 60 seconds after each.

MODIFIED BICYCLE KICK

Targets: Obliques, Rectus Abdominis

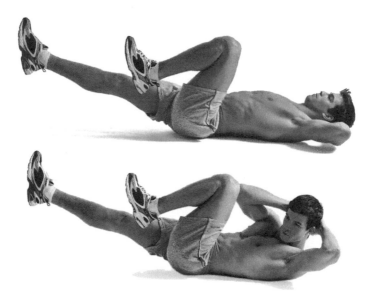

1 Lie on the floor with your hands behind your head, your right leg straight and off the floor. Bend your left leg so your knee is pulled toward your chest.

2 Lift your shoulder blades off the floor and take a count of two to touch your right elbow to your left knee. Pause, lower your elbow and shoulder blades back to the floor (again to a count of two), then immediately repeat the move on the other side—bringing your left elbow to your right knee and straightening your left leg.

3 Complete 15 repetitions on each side and then immediately do a set of 30 conventional crunches.

REVERSE CRUNCH

Targets: Rectus Abdominis

1. Lie faceup on the floor with your arms straight above you or braced on the sides of a doorway. Bend your knees and lift your heels off the floor and toward your butt.

2. Roll your hips up, bringing your knees toward your chest. As your lower back rises off the floor, straighten your legs, point your toes to the ceiling, and lift your hips. Pause, then slowly reverse the motion. Do 20 repetitions.

ROLL UP

Targets: Rectus Abdominis

1. Lie faceup on the floor with your legs straight and your arms at your sides.

2. Push your heels into the ground and slowly lift your shoulders and back off the floor. Pause when your upper body is perpendicular to the floor, then slowly lower your body to a count of five. Perform 10 repetitions.

THE 20-MINUTE WORKOUT

Sculpt Olympian Legs

The exercises in this circuit will help you build overall leg strength, flexibility, and endurance. If you're a beginner or haven't worked out in six months, do the moves as your lower-body workout and use only your body weight for each exercise. If you already work your legs weekly, incorporate these exercises into the beginning of your workout, but keep the weight light—5- or 10-pound dumbbells, for instance. Do the workout two or three times a week, with at least a day of rest between sessions. Perform three sets of 10 to 14 repetitions of each move; for the stepups, that means 10 to 14 with each leg.

FRONT STEPUP

Targets: Quadriceps, Hamstrings, Gluteals
Time: 5 Minutes

1. The step should be high enough that your thigh is parallel to the floor when your foot is on the step.

2. Place your left foot on the step and push yourself up until your left leg is straight. Your right foot doesn't need to rest on the step.

3. Step back down, right foot first, followed by your left.

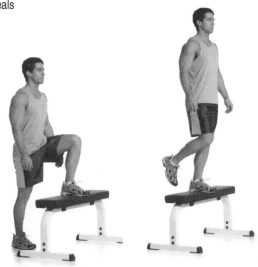

LATERAL STEPUP

Targets: Groin, Quadriceps, Hamstrings, Gluteals, Calves
Time: 5 Minutes

1. Use a step that's about 12 inches high.

2. Follow the same procedure as for the Front Stepup, but stand sideways next to the step instead of facing it.

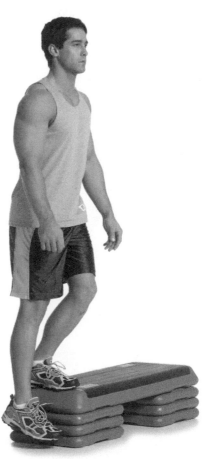

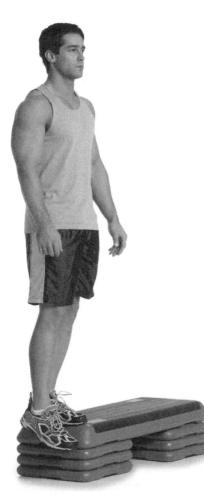

TRAINER'S TIPS

- Stand as straight as possible. This minimizes stress on the lower back and legs.

- Be certain to do the same number of repetitions for each foot. You can either alternate legs or complete a given number with one side, then switch to the other.

BELT SQUAT

Targets: Quadriceps, Hamstrings, Gluteals, Outer Thighs
Time: 5 Minutes

1 Stand with your hands behind your head and your knees slightly bent. Position a bungee cord just above your knees and push out as you squat.

2 Keep your body as upright as possible throughout the movement, and lower yourself until your thighs are parallel to the floor; then return to a standing position.

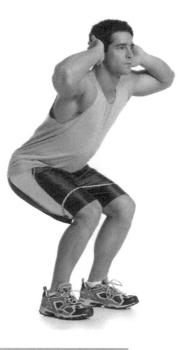

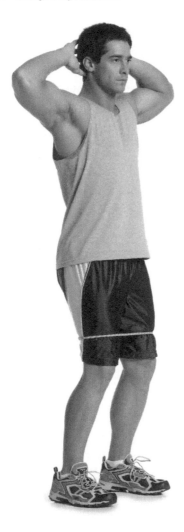

TRAINER'S TIP

Pushing out on the bungee cord with your outer-thigh muscles forces your adductors (inner-thigh muscles) to work harder to keep you stabilized.

BALL SQUAT

Targets: Quadriceps, Hamstrings, Gluteals, Inner Thighs
Time: 5 Minutes

1 Stand with your hands behind your head and your knees slightly bent. Hold a medicine ball or a basketball between your knees.

2 Keep your upper body as straight as possible and lower yourself until your thighs are parallel to the floor, then return to a standing position.

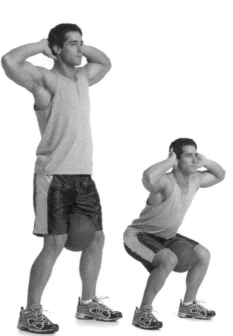

TRAINER'S TIP

Squeezing the ball with your adductors makes your abductors (outer thigh muscles) work overtime to help with your balance.

THE ULTIMATE POWER MOVE

If you aren't doing squats in your workout, then you don't have a workout. Squats shape the body and develop performance power—they're easy to learn and produce quick, dramatic results in both muscle size and strength.

To get the most out of each and every squat you do, focus on squatting deeper. The key is to descend until your thighs are parallel to the floor, while still keeping your heels on the floor and maintaining the natural arch in your lower back. This deeper squat builds muscle faster and is safer for your knees than a squat in which you stop before your thighs are parallel to the floor. When you cut a squat short like that, you turn your knees into brakes and you know what happens to brakes: They wear out.

⏱ THE 20-MINUTE WORKOUT

Lower-Body Beach Blast

Next time you head to the beach, you can get a great lower-body workout before you brave the waves and bathe in the sun. How? The secret is written in the sand. Sand provides less stability, making the simplest movements much harder. Don't go for the compacted sand near the water, which is too hard on the ankles. Find a soft, flat area, lose the shoes, and do two sets of each exercise, with a minute of rest between exercises. Repeat the circuit, reapply your sunscreen, and enjoy the rest of your day at the beach!

SHUTTLE RUN

Targets: Quadriceps, Calves, Hamstrings, Gluteals
Time: 5 Minutes

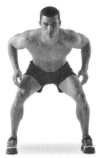
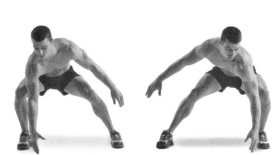

1 Make three parallel lines in the sand, 5 yards apart. Straddle the middle line with your knees slightly bent and your arms bent so your hands are in front of your thighs.

2 Move to your right and bend at the knees to touch the line with your right hand, then run to the left and touch the far left line with your left hand.

SAND SKIP

Targets: Quadriceps, Calves, Hamstrings, Gluteals
Time: 5 Minutes

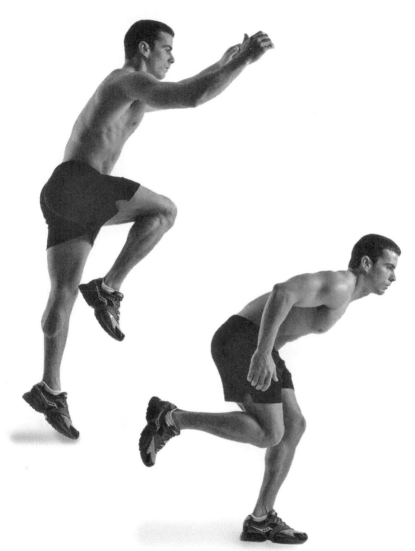

1 Skip forward so that you're jumping and landing on the same foot.

2 Work on leaping as high as possible by driving your knee upward as you push off the ground with your opposite foot. Do five skips on each leg.

SQUAT JUMP

Targets: Quadriceps, Calves, Hamstrings, Gluteals
Time: 5 Minutes

1. Stand with your feet slightly more than shoulder-width apart and your fingers laced behind your head.

2. Bend at the knees to lower yourself until your thighs are at least parallel to the sand, then jump up as high as you can.

3. Sink directly into the next squat without pausing. Do a total of five repetitions.

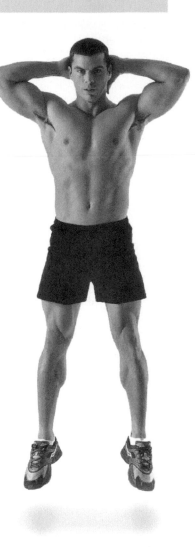

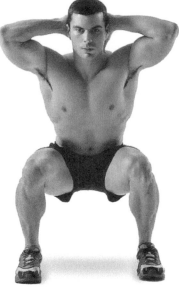

TRAINER'S TIP

Don't have a beach handy? You can still do the workout, but take care to protect your knees. Try to do these moves on a carpeted or padded surface; a wooden aerobics studio is ideal.

JUMP AND STICK

Targets: Quadriceps, Calves, Hamstrings, Gluteals
Time: 5 Minutes

1 Stand with your feet about shoulder-width apart, hands beside your thighs.

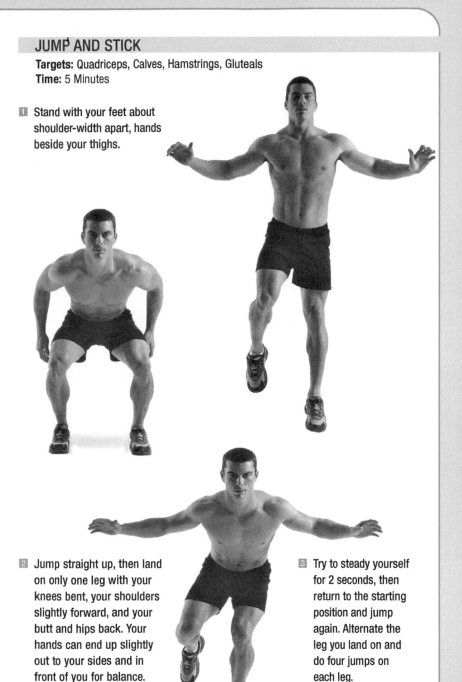

2 Jump straight up, then land on only one leg with your knees bent, your shoulders slightly forward, and your butt and hips back. Your hands can end up slightly out to your sides and in front of you for balance.

3 Try to steady yourself for 2 seconds, then return to the starting position and jump again. Alternate the leg you land on and do four jumps on each leg.

Balancing Act

Build Lower-Body Endurance

To truly excel in your sport of choice, you need balance, endurance, and strength. Whether you're racing down the soccer field or reaching for that seemingly impossible tennis shot, the ability to balance on a single leg, quickly change direction, and start and stop your motion with the snap of a finger is definitely an asset. Here's a circuit that will improve your balance and quicken your step. Warm up for 5 minutes, then do these exercises, with only a minute of rest after each.

SINGLE-LEG BALANCE SQUAT

Targets: Quadriceps, Gluteals

1 Stand on a block or step (start with one that's about 6 inches high) and move one foot off the edge.

2 Bend the knee of the supporting leg so that the nonsupporting foot brushes the floor. Hold that position for 3 to 5 seconds, and then stand back up.

TRAINER'S TIP

When you can comfortably perform 20 balance squats, it's time to up the stakes and make this move more challenging—increase the height of the block (or step) to further develop your balance, endurance, and coordination.

SINGLE-LEG SKI SQUAT

Targets: Quadriceps, Gluteals

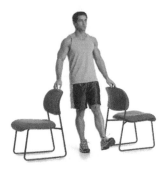

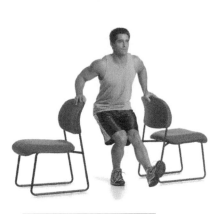

1. Stand on one leg, and place the other leg in front of you with your heel about 6 inches above the floor.

2. Squat down until the thigh of your back leg is almost parallel to the floor. Do 10 repetitions. Rest 15 seconds, then switch legs.

TRAINER'S TIP

If you're struggling to keep your balance, use two sturdy chairs for support until you feel comfortable with the move.

DOUBLE-LEG SKI SQUAT

Targets: Quadriceps, Gluteals

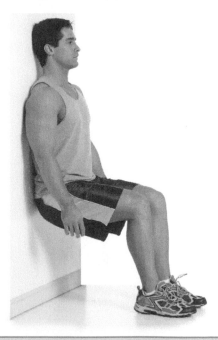

1. Lean against a wall, with your feet about 2 feet away from it and shoulder-width apart.

2. Bend your knees slightly and hold that position for 5 to 10 seconds. Bend deeper and hold.

3. Repeat until you've hit five different positions; go as low as you can without losing your balance. Work up to 30 seconds in each position.

Isoexplosion

2 Power Moves for Total-Body Training

You live in the real world; you're going to miss some workouts. But when there's no equipment at hand, you can rely on isoexplosive training. Using only your body weight to maintain muscle, you'll be able to work out when you're on the road, stuck in the office, or just unable to find your dumbbells. Try these two exercises for an intense full-body workout—anytime, anywhere. Do four or five sets of six to eight repetitions, alternating between exercises and resting 30 seconds between sets.

ISOEXPLOSIVE PUSHUP

Targets: Chest, Triceps, Shoulders, Abdominals

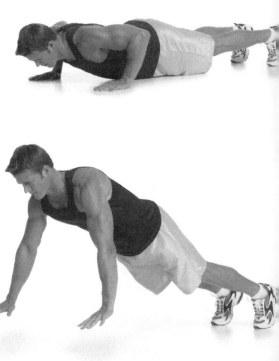

1. Get into a pushup position, hands slightly wider than and in line with your shoulders. Your body should form a straight line from your shoulders to your ankles.

2. Keep your back flat and lower your body until your upper arms are lower than your elbows. Pause, holding the "down" position for 4 seconds.

3. Forcefully thrust yourself upward as high as you can, so that your hands leave the floor. Catch yourself and repeat.

ISOEXPLOSIVE SQUAT

Targets: Quadriceps, Gluteals

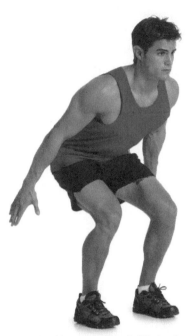

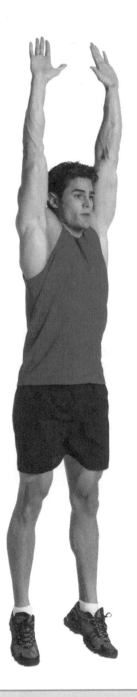

1 Stand with your knees slightly bent and your feet shoulder-width apart.

2 Slowly lower your body as if you were sitting back into a chair, keeping your back in its natural alignment, until the fronts of your thighs are parallel to the floor, or lower. Pause, holding the "down" position for 4 seconds. Jump as high as you can, then repeat.

ISOEXPLOSIVE BURN

To get the most out of these isoexplosive moves, hold the "down" position of each exercise for 4 seconds, which eliminates the elasticity in your muscles. When you explode upward, your muscle fibers will be forced to work maximally, without weights.

The 22-Minute Total-Body Plan

Sculpt Your Body with 16 Essential Weight-Free Moves

You want to get back into shape, right? But between long hours at work, business travel, and weekends spent frantically shuttling the kids from soccer practice to dance class to dentist's office, does anyone ever make it to the gym anymore? Here's a comprehensive, total-body workout you can do anytime, and just about any-where—hotel room, home gym, backyard, or even in the comfort of your living room.

Daily Stretches

Spend 10 minutes warming up with the eight stretches below every day before your total-body workout. Hold each position for 10 seconds.

The Workout

Do the routines on alternating days. For example, do Workout A on Monday, Workout B on Wednesday, and then Workout A again on Friday. The next week, do the oppo-site, with Workout B on Monday, A on Wednesday, and B again on Friday (see chart on following page). If you're a beginner, start off with five repetitions of each exercise the first week and gradually increase

the reps to 20. Do this slowly and carefully—don't push yourself too hard at first. When you're able to do 10 reps of each exercise, the workout should take 8 to 12 minutes to com-plete. The stretches should take about 10 minutes. Total workout time: 22 minutes.

Daily Stretches

Upper-Back Stretch (p.22)
Chest Stretch (p.23)
Shoulder and Neck Stretch (p.24)
Posterior Shoulder Stretch (p.25)
Lying Iliotibial-Band Stretch (p.28)
Modified Hurdler Stretch (p.29)
Groin Stretch (p.30)
Calf Stretch (p.30)

Workout A

EXERCISE	BEGINNER REPS	INTERMEDIATE REPS	ADVANCED REPS
Donkey kick (p.94)	5	10	20
Dive-bomber pushup (p.69)	5	10	20
Dirty dog (p.92)	5	10	20
Lunge (p.90)	5	10	20
Side straddle hop (p.94)	5	10	20
Back extension (p.74 and p.75)	5	10	20
Wide pushup (p.67)	5	10	20
Side crunch (p.86)	5	10	20
Crunch (p.79)	5	10	20

Workout B

EXERCISE	BEGINNER REPS	INTERMEDIATE REPS	ADVANCED REPS
Pushup (p.64)	5	10	20
Crunch (p.79)	5	10	20
Lunge (p.90)	5	10	20
Steam engine (p.88)	5	10	20
Elbow-to-knee crunch (p.87)	5	10	20
Prone flutter kick (p.76)	5	10	20
Hip adduction (p.93)	5	10	20
Side leg raise (p.91)	5	10	20
Diamond pushup (p.66)	5	10	20

The All-Day Workout

Build Strength and Flexibility Anytime, Anywhere

We all have time to exercise. It's the prep work that kills us. Gather your gear, drive to the gym, navigate the reception desk and locker room, warm up, cool down, stretch, shower, dress, and drive home—you invest more time accommodating exercise than actually working out. But we've found plenty of exercises you can do without all that wasted time. These moves take only moments—pumping you up or calming you down—and will contribute to your overall strength, flexibility, posture, and muscle. Best of all, they fit into the pockets of time hidden throughout the day—when you're between tasks at work, walking the dog, or getting ready for bed. On the busiest day of your life, you'll still have time to squeeze all of them in.

LYING VACUUM

Targets: Obliques, Transverse Abdominis

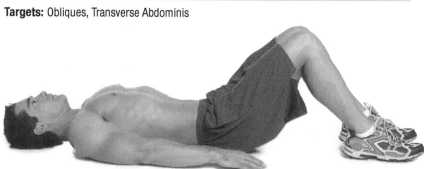

■ Lie on your back in bed and try to suck your belly button all the way back to your spine. While you're at it, try to tighten up the muscles on the sides of your midsection, too. Hold for 10 seconds while you take shallow breaths. Try it three times.

BRIDGE

Targets: All Mid-body Muscles

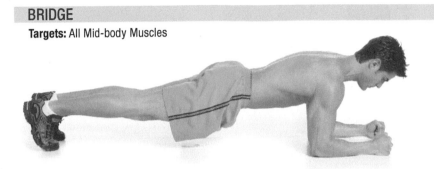

■ Lie facedown on the floor (on a rug or mat) and prop yourself up so your weight is on your toes, forearms, and hands. Your body should form a straight line from head to heels. Don't let your chest or stomach sag toward the floor. You have to tighten all your muscles to hold this position, with your abs and the muscles between your shoulder blades doing the hardest work. Again, hold 10 seconds while breathing, and do three repetitions.

WORK YOUR ABS BEFORE BREAKFAST

When you wake up in the morning, your abs are about as visible as they're going to be all day. So take advantage: Do these these abdominal exercises as soon as you wake up—you don't even have to get out of bed to do the Lying Vacuum (left).

TOWEL STRETCH

Targets: Shoulders, Triceps

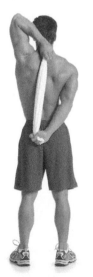

■ Grab the ends of the towel with your left hand behind your head and your right hand at the middle of your back. Gently pull down with your right hand until you feel a good stretch in your left shoulder and triceps. Hold for 15 to 30 seconds. Then pull up with your left hand until you feel a stretch in your right shoulder, and hold that for 15 to 30 seconds. Repeat two or three times, slowly going from one stretch to the other. Reverse hand positions and repeat two or three more times.

SHOWER AND STRETCH

Do this stretch right after you get out of the shower and towel off. It will help combat the tightness that develops in your shoulders when you hunch over a keyboard all day.

WALKING LUNGE

Targets: Quadriceps, Gluteals, Hamstrings

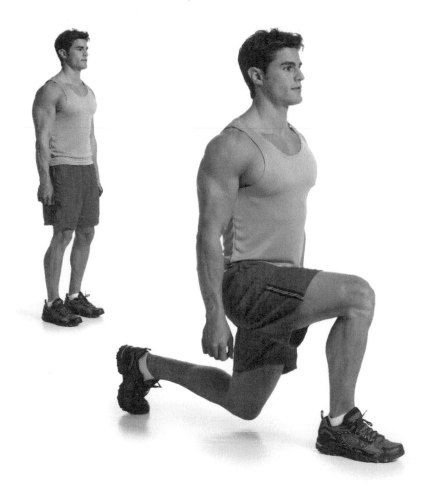

1 Lunge forward with your right leg, and walk forward with your left leg into another lunge step, making sure to that your right foot is directly under your front knee when in the lunged position. Do a set of walking lunges for 20 feet or so, then turn around and do another set.

THE ANYTIME LUNGE

You can work the stabilizing muscles in your calves, inner and outer thighs, and midsection by lunging instead of walking a few times a day. Do a few lunges in the morning while walking your dog, or on your way to the bathroom. You can even do lunging laps around your living room while watching your favorite television show—just make sure no one sees you.

HORSE STANCE

Targets: Legs, Hips, Ankles

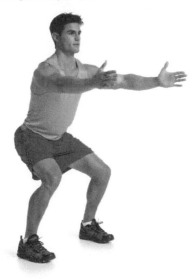

■ Stand with your feet shoulder-width apart and pointing forward. Keeping your head and back straight, squat down by bending your knees and extend your arms out in front of you, palms facing each other. Hold for up to 60 seconds, then shift to the Bow-and-Arrow Stance.

BOW-AND-ARROW STANCE

Targets: Legs, Hips

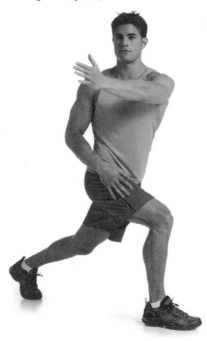

■ Stand with your legs a little more than shoulder width apart and extend your right foot forward. Place your right hand on your right thigh and reach your left arm across your chest. Hold for up to 60 seconds, return to the Horse Stance for 60 seconds, then repeat the Bow-and-Arrow Stance in the opposite direction for 60 seconds.

TRAINER'S TIP

The two stances shown on this page come from the world of martial arts; fighters use them to build strength and stamina in their lower bodies. These two are particularly beneficial for the muscles surrounding your knees, as they increase their stability.

HIP FLEXOR STRETCH

Targets: Hips

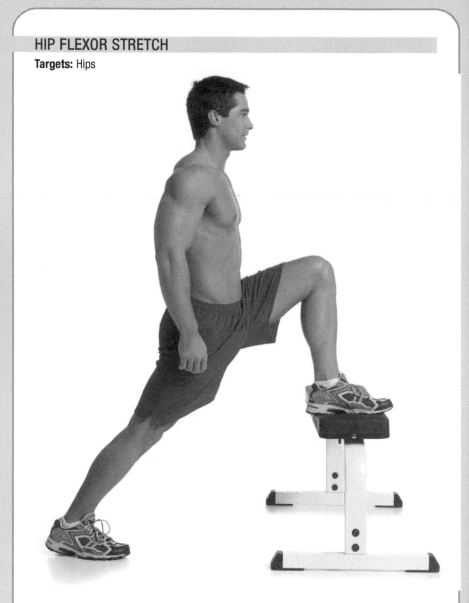

■ Plant your left foot on an elevated surface like a bench, a step, a chair, or even a fire hydrant. Lean toward it, bending your left leg while keeping your right leg straight. Feel the stretch on the front of your right hip. Hold for 30 seconds, then switch legs.

TRAINER'S TIP

Stretch your hip flexors whenever you have a chance. These muscles, which sit on the front of your pelvis, can become shortened and tightened from a full day of sitting.

PART III:
The Exercises

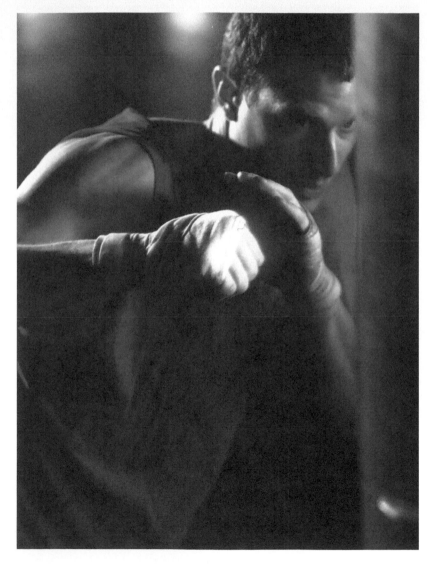

Chest, Back and Arms

Essential upper-body exercises for total-body strength and fitness

PUSHUP

■ **Targets:** Chest, Triceps, Shoulders

1 Get into pushup position—your hands set slightly wider than and in line with your shoulders—with your arms straight and your back flat.

2 Lower your body until your chest nearly touches the floor. Pause, then push yourself back up to the starting position.

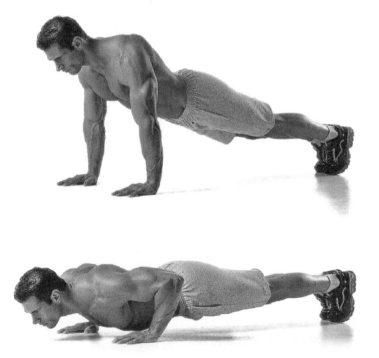

ONE-HANDED PUSHUP

■ **Targets:** Chest, Triceps, Shoulders

1 Spread your legs as wide as possible and move your arm toward the center of your body as shown.

2 Lower your body until your chest nearly touches the floor. Pause, then push yourself back up to the starting position.

TRAINER'S TIP

If you're having trouble doing the One-Handed Pushup, put your hand on an elevated surface, such as a chair. This reduces the percentage of body weight you have to lift, making the exercise easier.

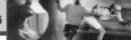

DIAMOND PUSHUP

■ **Targets:** Chest, Triceps, Shoulders

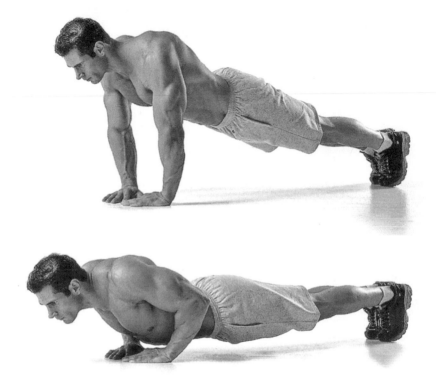

1 Get into traditional pushup position, but place your hands directly under your chest with your index fingers and thumbs spread and touching—that's the diamond.

2 Lower your body until your chest nearly touches your hands. Pause, then push your body back up to the starting position.

TRAINER'S TIP

To reap the most benefits from all your pushup pursuits, make sure to keep your back flat and your pelvis tucked in throughout the movement.

WIDE PUSHUP

■ **Targets:** Chest, Triceps, Shoulders

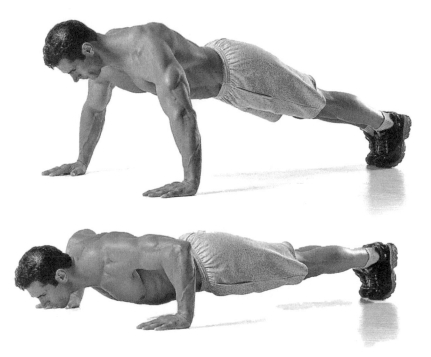

1 Get into pushup position, but place your hands about 5 inches wider than and in line with your shoulders.

2 Keeping your back flat, lower your body until your chest nearly touches the floor. Pause, then return to the starting position.

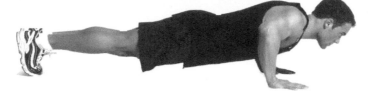

ROTATION PUSHUP

■ **Targets:** Chest, Triceps, Upper Back, Rear Shoulders

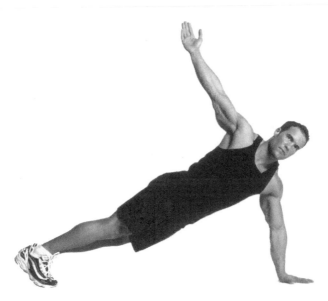

1 From the down position of a traditional pushup, raise your body. Reach your right hand toward the ceiling while twisting your torso to the right.

2 Lower your arm, and then slowly lower your body, rotating your torso back so that your chest is facing the floor. Repeat on other side.

PUSHUP POWER

Do you know how much of your own body weight you lift when doing a pushup? The answer might surprise you. At the top position of the pushup (when your arms are extended), you're supporting about 65 percent of your body weight. At the bottom position (when your upper arms are parallel to the floor), you're pressing about 75 percent of your body weight. That's not so bad when you think of how much you probably bench press at the gym.

DIVE-BOMBER PUSHUP

■ **Targets:** Chest, Front Deltoids, Triceps

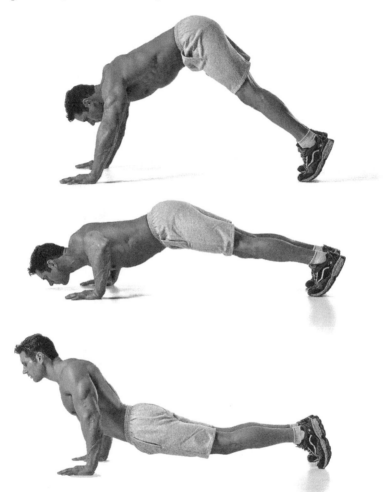

1. Get into a traditional pushup position, but place your hands slightly wider than and in front of your shoulders, in line with your ears. Raise your hips and move your feet forward as far as possible, without bending your back or legs, and place your feet beyond shoulder-width apart.

2. Move your chest down and forward until it nearly touches the floor and your shoulders are even with your hands.

3. Pause, then push your hips down as you straighten your arms. Pause again, then reverse the movement until you've come back to the starting position.

STEPUP PUSHUP

■ **Targets:** Chest, Triceps, Rotator Cuffs

1 Position yourself in a traditional pushup position in front of a step or bottom stair.

2 Move your right hand onto the stair while keeping your back straight, then move your left hand onto the step. Hold this position for 2 seconds.

3 Remove your right hand from the step, returning it to the floor. Bring your other hand back down into the starting position. Repeat the entire sequence.

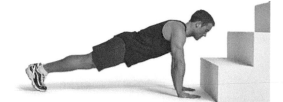

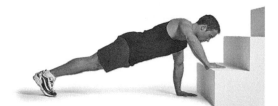

TRAINER'S TIP

Even though this pushup does not include the traditional pushup motion, it still provides a great upper-body workout by challenging your muscles to support your weight from uneven, unfamiliar angles.

STAGGERED PUSHUP

■ **Targets:** Chest, Triceps, Back, Abdominals

1 Position yourself in a traditional pushup posture. Keep your back straight, and place one hand 6 inches forward, so that it is in line with your ear.

2 Lower yourself until your chest is almost touching the floor, and slowly raise yourself to the starting position. Repeat by moving the other hand forward.

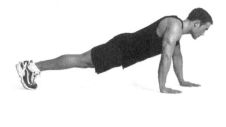

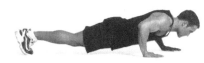

THREE-POINT PUSHUP

■ **Targets:** Chest, Triceps, Shoulders

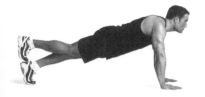

1 While in a traditional pushup position, place one foot on top of the other, so that the toe of the top foot is resting on the heel of the bottom foot. Your body is now resting on three points.

2 Keep your back straight and lower yourself until your chest is almost touching the floor. Slowly raise yourself to the starting position. Repeat with the other foot on top.

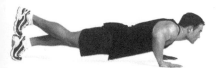

Y's, T's, and I's

If you are the athletic type, chances are you will strain or injure your rotator cuffs—a group of muscles and tendons that surround the top of the upper arm bone and enable your arm to move from your shoulder with force and speed—at some stage. These great exercises will help strengthen those muscles and prevent injury. The titles refer to the position of your arms and body as they form different letters of the alphabet. Do three sets of 10 repetitions of each.

Targets: Rotator Cuffs

1 Lie facedown on a bench and extend your arms in front of you to form a "Y." Keep your back straight and point your thumbs to the ceiling. Lift your arms toward the ceiling as much as you can by squeezing your shoulder blades. Although you won't move much, you'll feel a good stretch in those rotator cuffs. Lower your arms back to the starting position, and repeat.

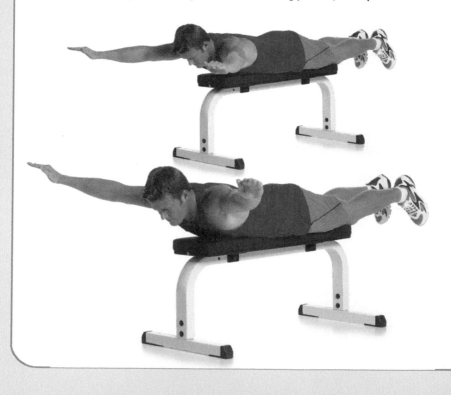

2 Next, stretch your arms, palms down, to either side of your body in the shape of a "T." Once again, try to lift your arms as high as you can by squeezing your shoulder blades. Lower your arms slowly, and repeat.

3 Finally, pull your arms to your sides, with palms facing in, and form the letter "I" with your body. Once more, raise your arms as high as you can. Slowly lower, and repeat.

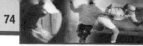

TOWEL CHEST FLY

■ **Targets:** Chest

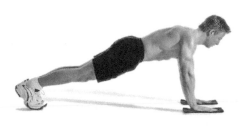

1. Place your hands on either a towel or a pair of socks. Assume the traditional top pushup position, with your hands close together underneath you and your feet hip-width apart.

2. Slide your hands out to your sides as you lower your body toward the floor. Slowly slide back up. Keep your elbows slightly bent throughout the movement, and make sure that your back is straight.

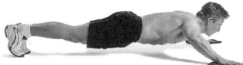

BACK EXTENSION I

■ **Targets:** Lower Back

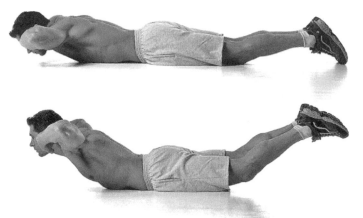

1. Lie facedown with your fingers behind your ears.

2. Simultaneously raise your upper body and legs off the floor as high as is comfortable. Pause, then slowly lower yourself back to the starting position and repeat.

BACK EXTENSION II

■ **Targets:** Lower Back

1. Lie facedown with your arms by your sides, a few inches away from your hips.

2. Simultaneously raise your upper body—including your arms—and your lower body off the floor as high as is comfortable. Pause, then slowly lower to the starting position, and repeat.

BATHROOM BREAKS TO SAVE YOUR BACK

Okay, so most of us spend hours on end sitting in uncomfortable desk chairs staring at computers, sealing business deals, and performing a myriad of other tasks. Nothing is easier than rounding your shoulders and resting your elbows on the desk while checking out a Web site. But you have to stay clear of such posture faux pas. The truth is, the best posture for sitting is one that changes frequently. If your job forces you to sit at a desk, leave your chair every 20 to 30 minutes to give your back intermittent breaks from the increased stress of sitting. An easy trick that will keep you out of that chair: Drink lots of water. Your bathroom breaks will give you an excuse to take your spine for a spin.

SUPERMAN

■ **Targets:** Lower Back

1 Lie facedown on the floor with your legs straight and your arms outstretched in front of you.

2 Simultaneously raise your upper body and legs off the floor as high as is comfortable. Pause, then slowly lower yourself back to the starting position and repeat.

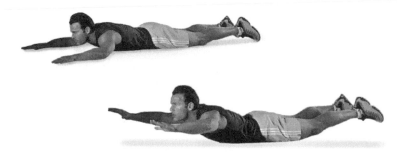

PRONE FLUTTER KICK

■ **Targets:** Hamstrings, Lower Back, Gluteals

1 Lie facedown on the floor with your legs straight and your arms in front of you. Raise your left leg off the floor as high as you can while your right leg remains stationary.

2 Pause, then lower your left leg to the starting position. Repeat with your right leg.

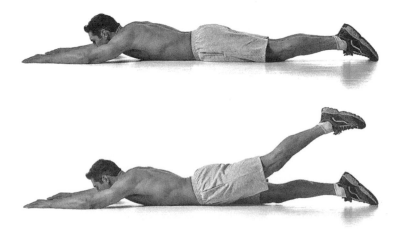

Abdominals

Crunch, twist, and slide your way to a strong, chiseled midsection

SHOULDER BRIDGE

■ **Targets:** Abdominals, Lower Back, Gluteals

1 Lie on your back with your legs bent and your feet flat on the floor.

2 Push your hips up so your weight rests on your shoulders. Your body should form a straight line from your knees to your shoulders.

3 Hold this position for 20 seconds, and gradually work your way up to one minute.

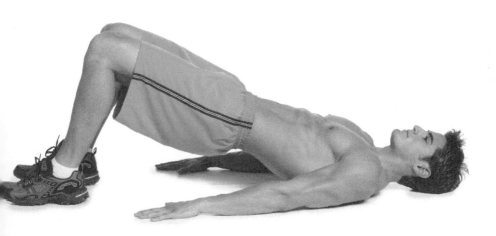

TRAINER'S TIP

As your lower-body strength improves, challenge your muscles in new ways by performing this variation: Straighten one leg and hold it up in the air. Start with your weaker leg in the air, and give equal time to both sides.

LYING VACUUM

■ **Targets:** Obliques, Transverse Abdominis

Lie on your back and contract your lower-abdominal muscles as if you're sucking your belly button all the way back to your spine. Hold for 10 seconds while you take shallow breaths.

DON'T HOLD YOUR BREATH

Although it's natural to want to hold your breath, it's important to breathe normally when performing isometric contractions like this one. If you're having trouble with this, place your hands on your abdomen and use your fingertips to gauge the intensity of the lower abdominal muscle contractions.

CRUNCH

■ **Targets:** Rectus Abdominis, Obliques

1 Lie on your back with your knees and hips bent about 90 degrees, and cross your arms.

2 Raise your upper body off the floor by crunching your rib cage toward your pelvis. Then lower yourself to the starting position.

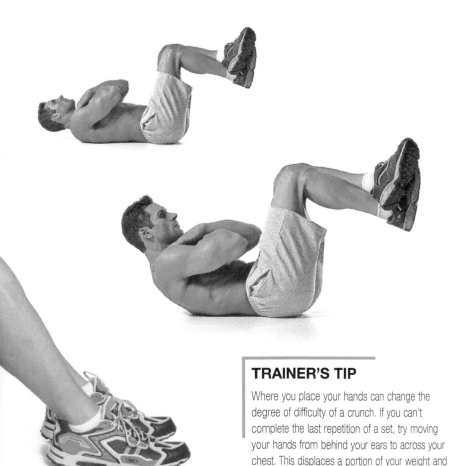

TRAINER'S TIP

Where you place your hands can change the degree of difficulty of a crunch. If you can't complete the last repetition of a set, try moving your hands from behind your ears to across your chest. This displaces a portion of your weight and may allow you to do one or two more crunches, to work the muscles a little longer.

LONG-ARM CRUNCH

■ **Targets:** Rectus Abdominis, Obliques

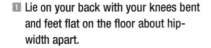

1 Lie on your back with your knees bent and feet flat on the floor about hip-width apart.

2 With your arms stretched over your head, exhale and slowly curl your head and torso toward your knees until your shoulder blades are off the floor. Use your upper abs to raise your rib cage toward your pelvis and lift your shoulder blades off the floor. Hold for a few seconds. Don't sit up fully; your lower back stays pressed to the mat.

3 Keeping your arms in line with your head, slowly lower yourself to the starting position, inhaling as you go. Use controlled motion; don't just drop to the floor.

TRAINER'S TIPS

• Make sure your shoulder blades come off the floor each time. Don't move just your head and neck.

• Pause at the top of the movement after you've exhaled.

• To align your head properly, put your tongue on the roof of your mouth when you do crunches, it will help reduce neck strain.

CRUNCH WITH HEEL PUSH

■ **Targets:** Rectus Abdominis, Obliques

1 Lie on your back with your knees bent and only your heels on the floor. Place your hands behind your ears, but avoid pulling your head forward.

2 Keeping your toes pointing up, slowly curl your head and torso toward your knees until your shoulder blades are off the floor. Hold for a few seconds, then slowly lower yourself to the starting position.

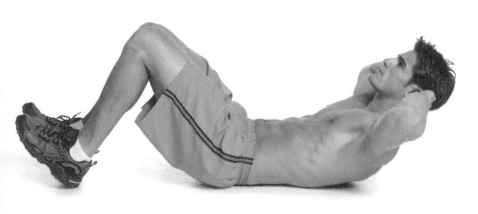

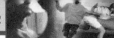

CROSS-LEGGED CRUNCH

■ **Targets:** Rectus Abdominis, Obliques

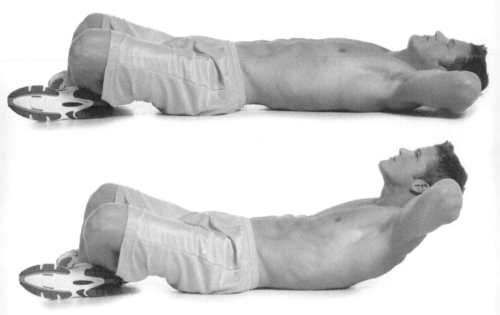

1 Lie on your back with your lower legs crossed on the floor. Hold your hands behind your ears and pull your elbows back as far as possible.

2 Slowly curl your head and torso toward your knees until your shoulder blades are off the floor. Hold for a few seconds, and slowly lower yourself to the starting position.

TRAINER'S TIP

For a more challenging exercise, start with your legs straight and suspended at a 45-degree angle to the floor. As you curl your upper body off the floor, simultaneously raise your legs until your feet point toward the ceiling. As you bring your head and shoulders back down to the floor, lower your legs back to a 45-degree angle.

TOWEL CRUNCH

■ **Targets:** Rectus Abdominis

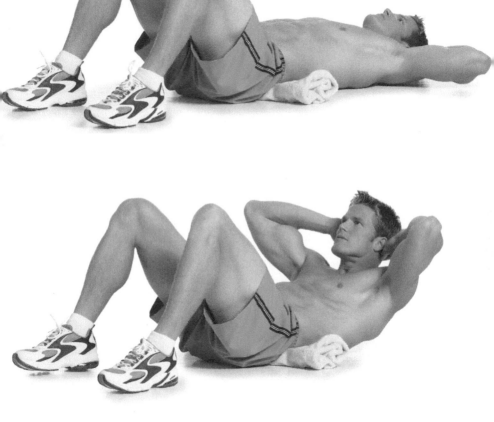

1 Sit on the floor with your knees bent, your feet flat on the floor, and your fingers behind your ears. Set a rolled-up towel under the arch of your lower back and lie back so your head rests on the floor.

2 Raise your head and shoulders and crunch your rib cage toward your pelvis.

3 Pause, then slowly return to the starting position.

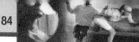

TWISTING LEGS-UP CRUNCH

■ **Targets:** Rectus Abdominis, Obliques

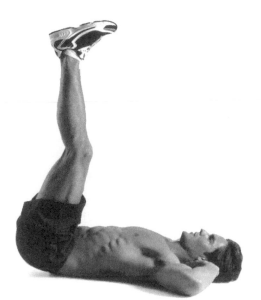

1 Lie on your back and raise your legs so that the soles of your feet point toward the ceiling.

2 Place your hands lightly behind your ears, elbows pointing out. Keeping your legs upright, slowly curl up and to the left.

3 Lower yourself and repeat to the right. Alternate from left to right throughout the set.

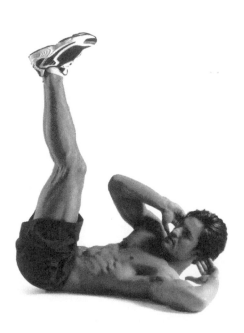

KNEE CRUNCH

■ **Targets:** Rectus Abdominis

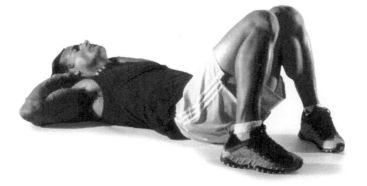

1. Lie on your back with your knees bent and together and your feet flat on the floor with your toes pointing in.

2. Place your hands behind your ears and lift your head and curl your shoulders up off the floor. Hold and then lower.

SIDE CRUNCH

■ **Targets:** Obliques

1 Lie on your right side and cross your right arm over your chest, resting your right hand on your left shoulder. Rest your left arm on your left side, with your palm down on your thigh.

2 Crunch your left armpit toward your left hip as you raise your legs off the floor. Pause, then return to the starting position. Repeat on the other side.

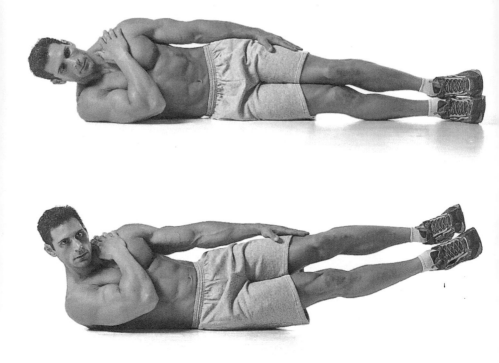

FEEL THE SQUEEZE

Here's a sure way to tell whether the exercise is effective: you feel a squeeze on the side of your stomach. Unlike the traditional crunch, this exercise works your obliques.

ELBOW-TO-KNEE CRUNCH

■ **Targets:** Rectus Abdominis, Obliques

1 Lie on your back, with your left foot flat on the floor and your right foot crossed over your left knee. Keep your arms folded over your chest.

2 Crunch your upper body, twisting it toward your right side. Touch your left elbow to your right thigh. Don't move just your elbow or shoulder—make sure you twist your whole torso toward your knee. Lower yourself slowly to the starting position. Repeat on the other side after switching legs.

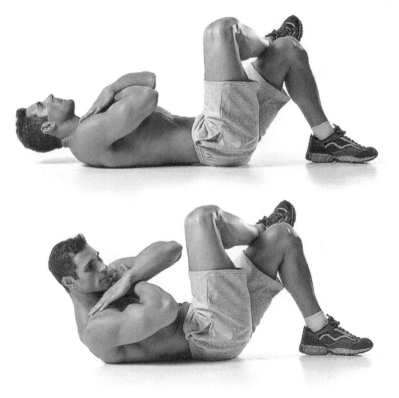

DON'T DO IT DAILY

Although it may be tempting to work your abs every day, they are just like any muscle group in your body: they need time to repair and rest. For best results, train them two to three times a week.

STEAM ENGINE

■ **Targets:** Hip Flexors, Entire Midsection

1 Stand with your hands cupping your ears from behind and your feet shoulder-width apart.

2 Bend and raise your right knee while you twist your left elbow toward your knee. Crunch your left shoulder toward your right hip to make contact between the elbow and the knee. Return to the standing position. Twist to the other side.

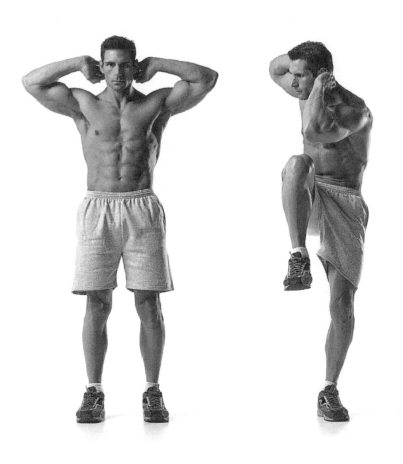

TOWEL SLIDE

■ **Targets:** Rectus Abdominis

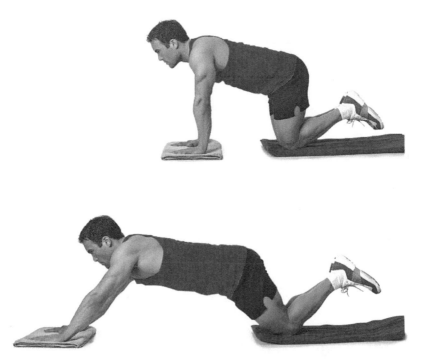

■ Kneel on a towel or mat on a tile or wooden floor. Put a towel on the floor in front of you and place your hands on it.

② Slide the front towel across the floor until your body is fully extended. Your body should look as if it's in a diving position. Slowly slide back up.

Legs

Build strong, supple muscles with this selection of lower-body exercises

THE LUNGE

■ **Targets:** Quadriceps, Gluteals, and Hamstrings

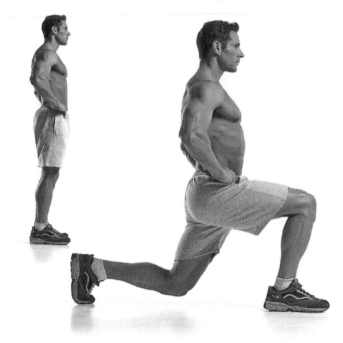

1 Stand with your hands on your hips and your feet hip-width apart.

2 Step forward with your right leg and lower your body until your right knee is bent 90 degrees and your left knee is almost touching the floor. Raise your body back to the starting position, and repeat with your left leg.

TRY IT IN REVERSE

To really strengthen your legs, try the lunge in reverse: Instead of moving forward as in the traditional lunge, step backward. How does it work? In a traditional lunge, your back leg gets the good stretch, while the front leg supports the movement. However, the reverse lunge forces your front leg to work throughout the entire exercise, increasing muscle use.

SIDE LEG RAISE

■ **Targets:** Outer Hips

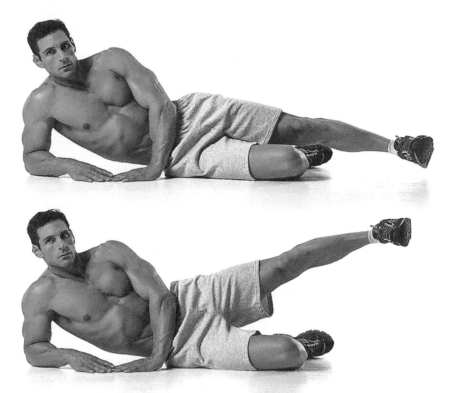

1. Lie on your right side while supporting yourself on your right elbow. Bend your right knee, but keep your left leg straight.

2. Leading with the heel, raise your left leg about 18 inches, and pause. Lower the leg to the starting position. After completing a set with your left leg, change sides and repeat with the other leg.

MAXIMIZE MUSCLE USE

Want to maximize your workout? Then do your lunges before the leg raises. Why? Lunges require balance and use small muscles that stabilize your body. These muscles get tired faster and therefore should be worked before moving onto exercises that don't require their use. That way, when you do those lunges, you won't be relying on overworked muscles to keep you stable.

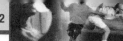
DIRTY DOG

■ **Targets:** Outer Hips

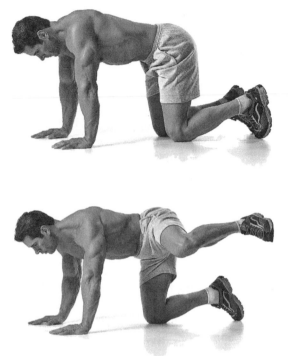

1 Get on your hands and knees, with your palms flat on the floor and your arms shoulder-width apart. While keeping your left leg bent, raise it out to the side from the hip.

2 Pause, then return your leg to the starting position. Repeat with the other leg.

STRONG ANKLES AND A QUICKER STEP

Improve ankle stability and increase agility with this tried and tested drill.

- Draw a line on the floor. Stand with your knees slightly bent, feet shoulder-width apart, hands in front of your body, and hips back. Bend your torso forward slightly so that you are balanced. Put your toes on the line.

- With one foot, step over the line and back repeatedly as fast as you can for 15 seconds. Tap your toes on the other side of the line and then return to the starting position. Repeat on the other side.

- Also, mix it up by stepping sideways, backwards, and back and forth with both feet.

HIP ADDUCTION

■ **Targets:** Inner Thighs

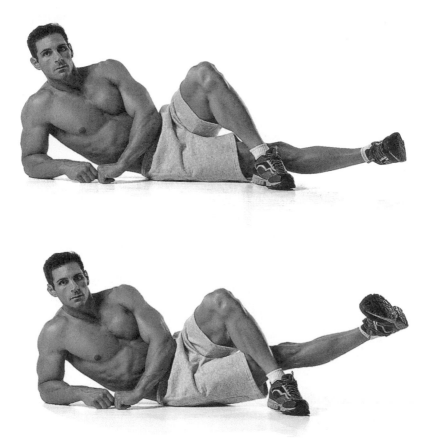

■ Lie on your right side, supporting your weight with your right elbow. With your right leg outstretched, place your left foot in front of your right knee, so that the left leg is bent.

■ Lift your right leg as high as you can toward the ceiling. You should feel a stretch in your inner thigh.

■ Slowly lower your leg back to the starting position. When you are done with a set, repeat with the other leg.

CURE YOUR CRAMPS

Ever overwork your legs so that they cramp up? Well, you may not have overworked them after all. Muscle cramps after a workout can be a sign of a deficiency. Your muscles need certain nutrients that can be depleted through exercise. Replace the lost potassium and magnesium in your body by grabbing a banana. Your legs will thank you.

SIDE STRADDLE HOP

■ **Targets:** Groin, Calves

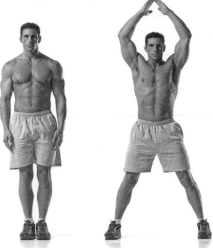

1 Stand with your feet together and arms hanging comfortably at your sides.

2 Jump and land with your feet just beyond shoulder-width apart while clapping your hands together overhead.

3 Jump back to the starting position, bringing your arms back down as well.

DONKEY KICK

■ **Targets:** Hamstrings, Hip Extensors

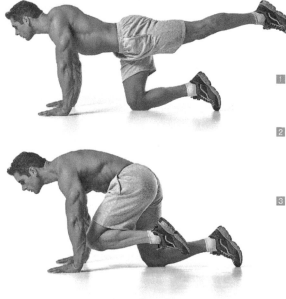

1 Get down on your hands and knees with your arms shoulder-width apart.

2 Balance your weight on your right leg and kick your left leg back and up as high as you comfortably can.

3 Finish by pulling your knee to your chest. Repeat with the other leg.

INDEX